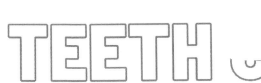

TEETH CHART

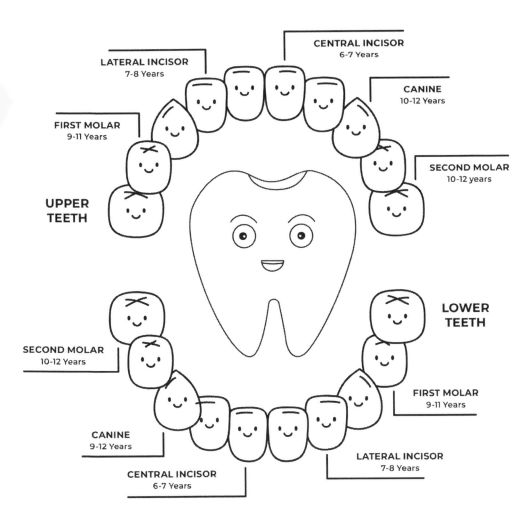

CENTRAL INCISOR
6-7 Years

LATERAL INCISOR
7-8 Years

CANINE
10-12 Years

FIRST MOLAR
9-11 Years

SECOND MOLAR
10-12 years

UPPER TEETH

LOWER TEETH

SECOND MOLAR
10-12 Years

FIRST MOLAR
9-11 Years

CANINE
9-12 Years

LATERAL INCISOR
7-8 Years

CENTRAL INCISOR
6-7 Years

HAPPY

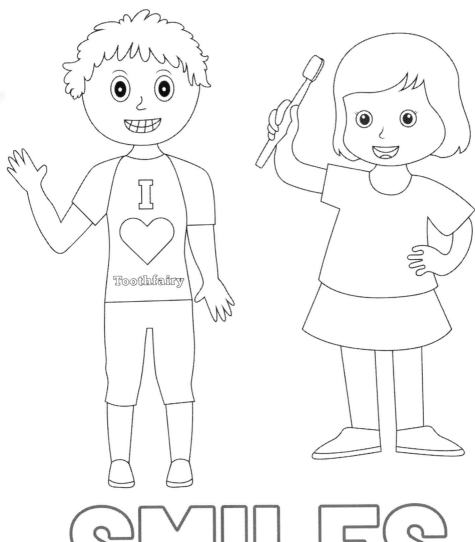

SMILES

SAY

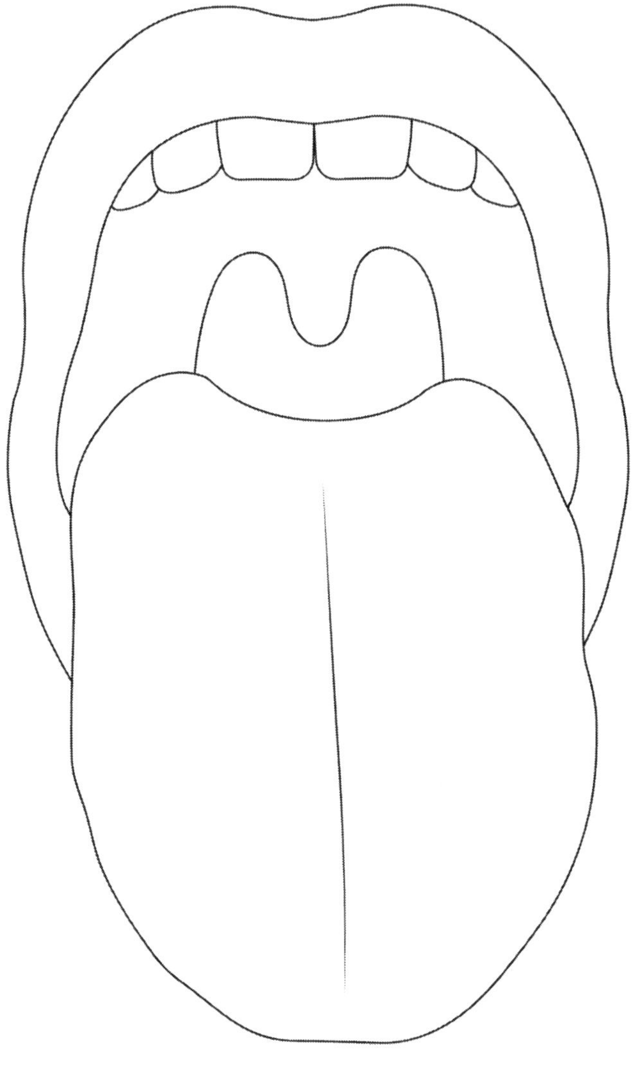

AAH

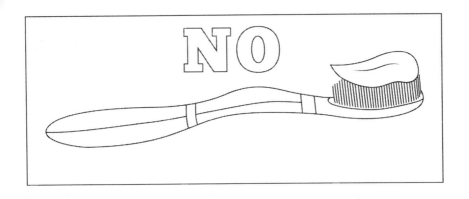

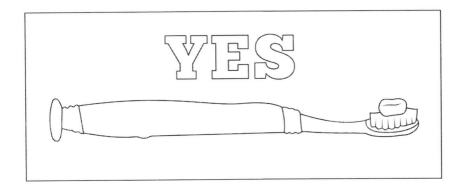

A PEA SIZED AMOUNT OF TOOTHPASTE IS ALWAYS BEST !

NO SUGAR BUGS FOR ME!

DECAY

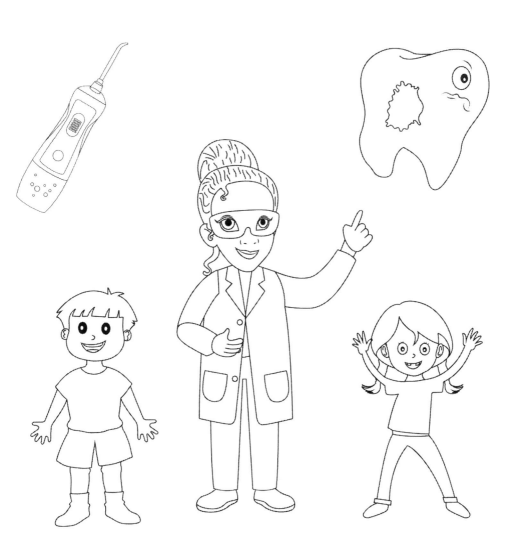

GO AWAY

HEALTHY

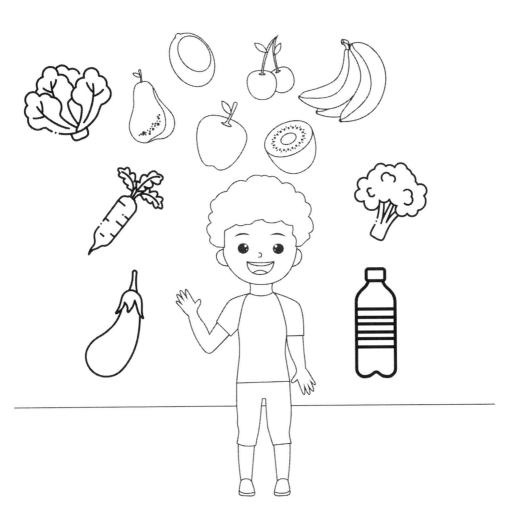

ME!

FIGHT GERMS IN YOUR MOUTH WITH BRUSHING, FLOSSING AND RINSING.

Streptococcus

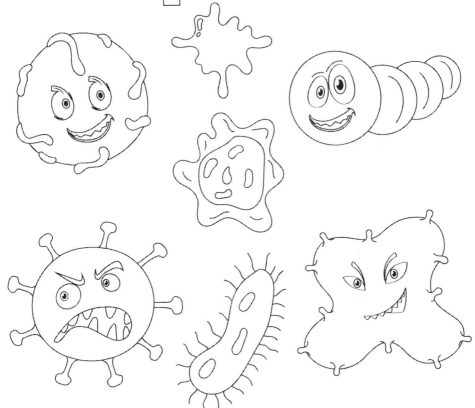

CAUSES
GINGIVITIS

PROTECT YOUR MOUTH

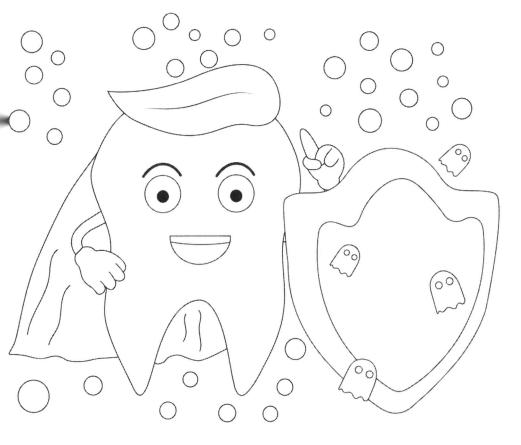

Brush 2x/day

Brush

Floss

Rinse

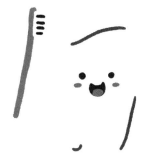

I LOVE

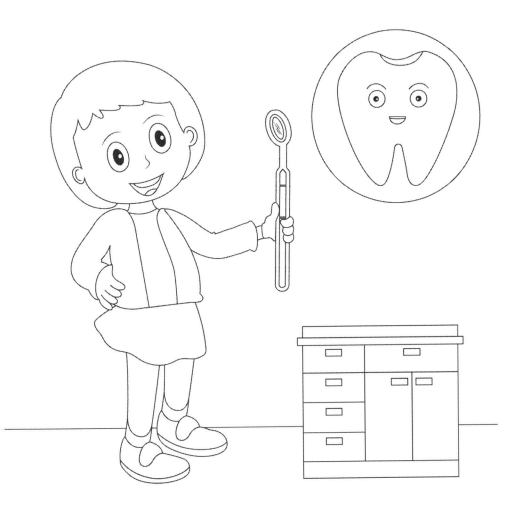

MY SMILE

FRUITS & VEGGIES MAKE
MY TEETH STRONG & HAPPY

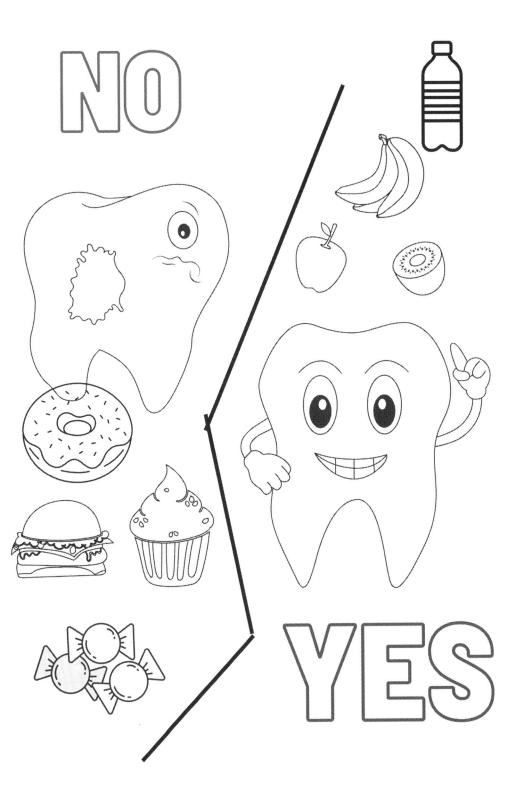

MORNING & NIGHT, BRUSH YOUR TEETH!

SAY NO TO PLAQUE !

BRUSH

2x a day

2 minutes

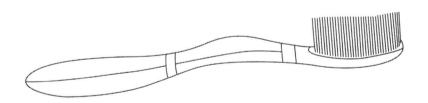

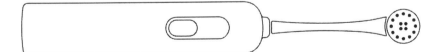

VISIT A DENTIST TWICE A YEAR !

DENTIST

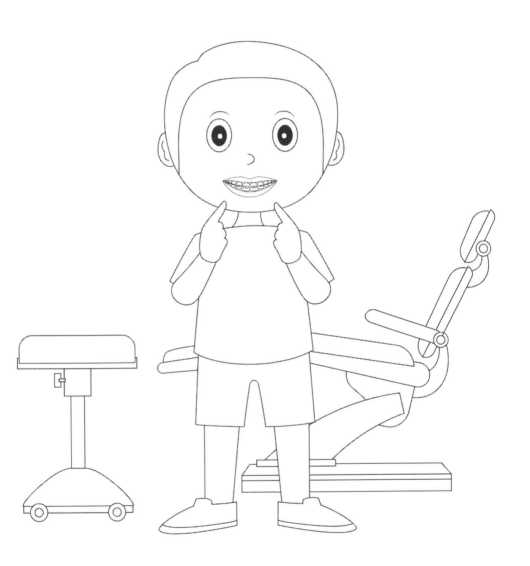

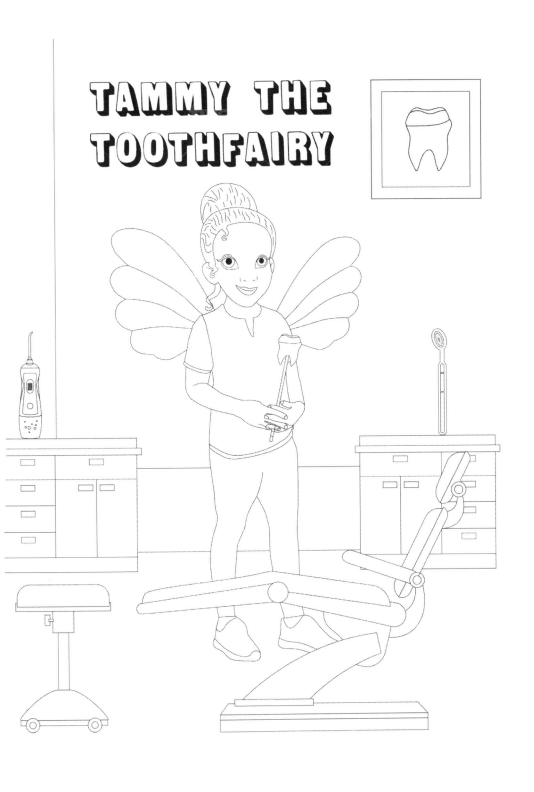

CHECKLIST

☐ **EAT HEALTHY**

☐ **BRUSH MY TEETH**

☐ **FLOSS MY TEETH**

☐ **RINSE MY MOUTH**

☐ **VISIT THE TOOTHFAIRY TWICE. A YEAR**

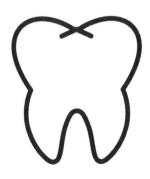

Made in the USA
Middletown, DE
14 October 2023

40620478R00018